Prostate Cancer Diet Cookbook For Men

Gerald Lea

Disclaimer

Please bear in mind that the information in this book is strictly educational. The data presented here is claimed to be credible and trustworthy. The author provides no implied or explicit assurance of accuracy for specific individual instances.

It is important that you consult with a skilled practitioner, such as your doctor, before initiating any diet or lifestyle changes. The information in this book should not be used in place of expert advice or professional assistance.

The author, publisher, and distributor fully disclaim any and all liability, loss, damage, or risk suffered by anybody who relies on the information in this book, whether directly or indirectly.

CONTENTS

Introduction

Welcome to the "Prostate Cancer Diet Cookbook for Men." In the pages that follow, we embark on a journey that goes beyond the traditional realms of a cookbook. This collection of recipes and guidance is crafted with a profound understanding of the critical role nutrition plays in maintaining and improving prostate health. Before delving into the culinary treasures that lie ahead, let's take a moment to explore why this book is not just a cookbook but a comprehensive guide to empower you on your path to a healthier, more resilient prostate.

The significance of nutrition in fostering overall well-being is indisputable, but its specific impact on prostate health is often underestimated. The prostate, a small gland with a big responsibility, is susceptible to various conditions, including cancer. As we unravel the complex relationship between diet and prostate health, it becomes evident that the food choices we make can significantly influence the risk of prostate-related issues.

Prostate cancer is one of the most common cancers affecting men worldwide. While various factors contribute to its development, scientific research increasingly points to the role of diet in either mitigating or exacerbating the risk. This chapter aims to demystify the link between nutrition and prostate cancer, highlighting the specific dietary components that can either serve as protective factors or potential contributors to the disease.

Through an exploration of epidemiological studies and clinical research, we shed light on the significance of adopting a prostate cancer diet. By understanding why certain foods are recommended and others discouraged, readers will gain valuable insights into the proactive steps they can take to reduce their risk of prostate cancer. This section serves as a compelling foundation for the transformative journey toward a healthier lifestyle.

Now that the groundwork is laid, it's time to introduce the heart of this book—the recipes and practical guidance that make up the Prostate Cancer Diet Cookbook for Men. This cookbook is not just a compilation of delicious and nutritious recipes; it is a tool designed to empower you to take control of your health through conscious, purposeful eating.

Each recipe in this collection is meticulously crafted to include ingredients that have been selected for their potential to support prostate health. From breakfast to dinner and everything in between, these recipes are more than just meals—they are a proactive step towards a healthier future. The cookbook is not merely a list of instructions on how to prepare a dish; it is a comprehensive resource that provides nutritional information, cooking tips, and a roadmap for incorporating these recipes into your daily life.

As you embark on this culinary journey, remember that this cookbook is more than just a guide to preparing meals; it is a companion on your path to better health. By embracing the principles outlined in this book and savoring the flavorful, prostate-friendly dishes within, you are not just nourishing your body but actively working towards a future of enhanced well-being and resilience.

So, let the pages ahead be a source of inspiration and empowerment as you explore the delectable intersection of nutrition and prostate health in the Prostate Cancer Diet Cookbook for Men. Your journey to a healthier, more vibrant life starts here.

Prostate Cancer Diet Cookbook For Men

Healthy Living At Your Fingertips

Chapter 1: Prostate Health Basics

The prostate gland is a crucial component of the male reproductive system, playing a pivotal role in both sexual function and urinary control. In this chapter, we will delve into the anatomy and function of the prostate gland, explore common prostate health concerns, and examine the intricate relationship between diet and the risk of prostate cancer.

Anatomy and Function of the Prostate Gland

The prostate gland is a walnut-sized organ located just below the bladder and in front of the rectum. It surrounds the urethra, the tube that carries urine from the bladder and semen from the reproductive system out through the penis. The primary function of the prostate is to produce a fluid that, when mixed with sperm from the testicles and fluids from other accessory glands, forms semen. This fluid provides nourishment and protection for the sperm, enhancing their viability and motility.

The prostate undergoes two significant growth phases in a man's life. The first phase occurs during puberty when the prostate doubles in size. The second phase begins around the age of 25 and continues throughout most of a man's life. This continuous growth can sometimes lead to issues such as benign prostatic hyperplasia (BPH), a non-cancerous enlargement of the prostate that can cause urinary symptoms.

Common Prostate Health Concerns

Several health issues can affect the prostate gland, ranging from benign conditions to more serious diseases. One of the most common concerns is BPH, which becomes increasingly prevalent with age and can result in symptoms like frequent urination, urgency, and difficulty starting or stopping the urinary stream.

Another significant concern is prostatitis, an inflammation of the prostate that can be caused by bacterial infections or other factors. Prostatitis can lead to discomfort, pain during urination, and other urinary symptoms. While often treatable with medication, prostatitis can significantly impact a man's quality of life.

Of greater concern is prostate cancer, one of the most prevalent cancers in men. Prostate cancer typically develops slowly and may not cause noticeable symptoms in its early stages. Regular screenings, including prostate-specific antigen (PSA) blood tests and digital rectal exams, are crucial for early detection. Treatment options for prostate cancer vary and may include surgery, radiation therapy, hormone therapy, or active surveillance.

The Link Between Diet and Prostate Cancer Risk

Mounting evidence suggests that diet plays a vital role in influencing the risk of developing prostate cancer. Various studies have explored the impact of dietary choices on prostate health, with a particular focus on the association between certain foods, nutrients, and the development of prostate cancer.

A diet rich in fruits and vegetables, especially those containing antioxidants such as lycopene (found in tomatoes) and cruciferous vegetables, has been linked to a lower risk of prostate cancer. Conversely, diets high in red and processed meats, as well as high-fat dairy products, may contribute to an increased risk.

Additionally, some studies have investigated the potential benefits of certain supplements, such as selenium and vitamin E, in reducing prostate cancer risk. However, the relationship between specific nutrients and prostate health remains complex, and further research is needed to establish clear guidelines.

Understanding the basics of prostate health, including its anatomy, common concerns, and the dietary factors influencing cancer risk, lays the foundation for a comprehensive approach to maintaining a healthy prostate.

Chapter 2: The Prostate Cancer Diet Framework

An integral aspect of managing prostate health, particularly in the context of preventing or addressing prostate cancer, involves adopting a well-rounded and nutritious diet. In this chapter, we will explore the essential nutrients crucial for prostate health, delineate foods that should be included in a prostate cancer diet, and discuss the importance of balancing macronutrients for overall well-being.

Key Nutrients for Prostate Health

Several key nutrients have been identified for their potential role in supporting prostate health and mitigating the risk of prostate cancer. Understanding and incorporating these nutrients into one's diet can be a proactive approach to maintaining optimal prostate function. Some of the key nutrients include:

1. **Lycopene:** Found abundantly in tomatoes and other red fruits, lycopene is a powerful antioxidant that has been associated with a reduced risk of prostate cancer.
2. **Cruciferous Vegetables:** Vegetables such as broccoli, cauliflower, Brussels sprouts, and kale contain compounds like sulforaphane, which have shown anti-cancer properties.
3. **Omega-3 Fatty Acids:** Found in fatty fish, flaxseeds, and walnuts, omega-3 fatty acids have anti-inflammatory properties that may contribute to prostate health.
4. **Selenium:** This trace mineral is present in nuts, seeds, and certain seafood. Some studies suggest that selenium may have a protective effect against prostate cancer.
5. **Vitamin D:** Adequate levels of vitamin D, obtained through sunlight exposure and dietary sources like fatty fish and fortified foods, have been linked to a lower risk of aggressive prostate cancer.
6. **Zinc:** Found in abundance in meat, dairy, and nuts, zinc is essential for prostate function, and a deficiency may contribute to prostate-related issues.

Foods to Embrace and Foods to Limit

Building a prostate-friendly diet involves making conscious choices about the foods we consume. Embracing a variety of nutrient-dense foods while limiting those that may pose a risk is crucial. Here are some dietary recommendations:

Foods to Embrace:
1. **Colorful Fruits and Vegetables:** Aim for a diverse range of fruits and vegetables to ensure a broad spectrum of vitamins, minerals, and antioxidants.
2. **Fatty Fish:** Include sources of omega-3 fatty acids like salmon, mackerel, and trout in your diet.
3. **Whole Grains:** Opt for whole grains such as brown rice, quinoa, and whole wheat for fiber and essential nutrients.
4. **Nuts and Seeds:** Incorporate a variety of nuts and seeds, which provide healthy fats, zinc, and selenium.
5. **Green Tea:** Some studies suggest that the antioxidants in green tea may have a protective effect against prostate cancer.

Foods to Limit:
1. **Red and Processed Meats:** Limit the consumption of red and processed meats, as they have been associated with an increased risk of prostate cancer.
2. **High-Fat Dairy:** Choose low-fat or fat-free dairy options to reduce saturated fat intake.
3. **Sugary Foods and Beverages:** High intake of sugar has been linked to inflammation, which may contribute to cancer development.
4. **Processed Foods:** Minimize the consumption of processed foods that are often high in unhealthy fats, sodium, and additives.

Balancing Macronutrients for Optimal Well-being

In addition to focusing on specific nutrients and food choices, achieving a balance of macronutrients—carbohydrates, proteins, and fats—is essential for overall well-being. A well-balanced diet provides the necessary energy and nutrients for bodily functions, supports immune health, and helps maintain a healthy weight.
1. **Carbohydrates:** Choose complex carbohydrates such as whole grains, fruits, and vegetables over refined and processed options. These provide sustained energy and essential nutrients.
2. **Proteins:** Include lean protein sources like poultry, fish, beans, and tofu. Protein is crucial for muscle health and immune function.
3. **Fats:** Opt for healthy fats from sources like olive oil, avocados, nuts, and fatty fish. These fats support heart health and provide essential fatty acids.

Balancing macronutrients ensures that the body receives a comprehensive array of nutrients necessary for optimal functioning, helping to support overall health, including prostate health.

14-Day Meal Plan

Day 1:
- **Breakfast:** Vegetable and Tofu Scramble (Page 19)
- **Lunch:** Lentil and Vegetable Soup (Page 25)
- **Dinner:** Baked Lemon Herb Salmon (Page 37)
- **Smoothie:** Berry Blast Smoothie with Spinach (Page 81)

Day 2:
- **Breakfast:** Almond Butter Banana Smoothie Bowl (Page 19)
- **Lunch:** Quinoa Salad with Grilled Chicken (Page 26)
- **Dinner:** Eggplant and Chickpea Curry (Page 42)
- **Smoothie:** Green Tea and Mango Smoothie (Page 81)

Day 3:
- **Breakfast:** Sweet Potato Hash with Turkey Sausage (Page 20)
- **Lunch:** Grilled Portobello Mushroom Salad (Page 30)
- **Dinner:** Spaghetti Squash with Turkey Bolognese (Page 37)
- **Smoothie:** Pineapple and Kale Smoothie (Page 82)

Day 4:
- **Breakfast:** Greek Yogurt and Berry Smoothie (Page 21)
- **Lunch:** Broccoli and Cheddar Stuffed Baked Potatoes (Page 32)
- **Dinner:** Grilled Tofu and Vegetable Skewers (Page 43)
- **Smoothie:** Blueberry and Almond Milk Smoothie (Page 83)

Day 5:
- **Breakfast:** Oatmeal with Pecans and Dried Cranberries (Page 21)
- **Lunch:** Quinoa and Black Bean Burrito Bowl (Page 32)
- **Dinner:** Spinach and Mushroom Stuffed Chicken Breast (Page 44)
- **Smoothie:** Kiwi and Orange Smoothie (Page 86)

Day 6:
- **Breakfast:** Breakfast Burrito with Black Beans and Salsa (Page 22)
- **Lunch:** Mediterranean Chicken Salad (Page 33)
- **Dinner:** Cauliflower and Lentil Curry (Page 45)
- **Smoothie:** Banana and Peanut Butter Protein Smoothie (Page 84)

Day 7:
- **Breakfast:** Cottage Cheese and Pineapple Bowl (Page 23)
- **Lunch:** Barley and Vegetable Stir-Fry (Page 34)
- **Dinner:** Lemon Garlic Herb Grilled Chicken (Page 46)
- **Smoothie:** Carrot and Ginger Immunity Boosting Smoothie (Page 87)

Day 8:
- **Breakfast:** Whole Wheat English Muffin with Smoked Salmon (Page 23)
- **Lunch:** Shrimp and Quinoa Spring Rolls (Page 35)
- **Dinner:** Whole Wheat Pasta with Tomato and Basil (Page 46)
- **Smoothie:** Spinach and Pineapple Detox Smoothie (Page 84)

Day 9:
- **Breakfast:** Avocado Toast with Poached Egg (Page 16)
- **Lunch:** Caprese Sandwich with Whole Grain Bread (Page 35)
- **Dinner:** Zucchini Noodles with Pesto and Cherry Tomatoes (Page 47)
- **Smoothie:** Berry and Yogurt Popsicles (Page 73)

Day 10:
- **Breakfast:** Salmon and Cream Cheese Bagel (Page 17)
- **Lunch:** Brown Rice Bowl with Teriyaki Salmon (Page 29)
- **Dinner:** Beef and Vegetable Lettuce Wraps (Page 48)
- **Smoothie:** Watermelon and Mint Smoothie (Page 86)

Day 11:
- **Breakfast:** Quinoa Breakfast Bowl with Berries and Almonds (Page 14)
- **Lunch:** Grains and Legumes: Quinoa Pilaf with Mixed Vegetables (Page 49)
- **Dinner:** Grilled Vegetable and Chicken Kebabs (Page 38)
- **Smoothie:** Blueberry and Almond Milk Smoothie (Page 83)

Day 12:
- **Breakfast:** Chia Seed Pudding with Mango (Page 16)
- **Lunch:** Nuts and Seeds: Chia Seed Energy Balls (Page 62)
- **Dinner:** Spinach and Pineapple Detox Smoothie (Page 84)
- **Smoothie:** Kiwi and Orange Smoothie (Page 86)

Day 13:
- **Breakfast:** Whole Grain Pancakes with Walnuts (Page 18)
- **Lunch:** Dinner: Grilled Pineapple with Honey and Pistachios (Page 79)
- **Dinner:** Barley Risotto with Roasted Butternut Squash (Page 50)
- **Smoothie:** Carrot and Ginger Immunity Boosting Smoothie (Page 87)

Day 14:
- **Breakfast:** Blueberry and Greek Yogurt Parfait (Page 15)
- **Lunch:** Grains and Legumes: Wild Rice with Mixed Mushrooms (Page 55)
- **Dinner:** Baked Cod with Garlic and Herbs (Page 42)
- **Smoothie:** Avocado and Berry Smoothie (Page 85)

Breakfast

Quinoa Breakfast Bowl with Berries and Almonds

- **Total Time:** 20 minutes
- **Servings:** 2

Ingredients:
- 1 cup cooked quinoa
- 1 cup mixed berries (strawberries, blueberries, raspberries)
- 1/4 cup sliced almonds
- 2 tablespoons honey
- 1/2 teaspoon vanilla extract
- Greek yogurt (optional, for topping)

Directions:
1. In a bowl, combine cooked quinoa, mixed berries, sliced almonds, honey, and vanilla extract.
2. Mix well until ingredients are evenly distributed.
3. Divide the mixture into two bowls and top with a dollop of Greek yogurt if desired.
4. Drizzle with additional honey and sprinkle with extra almonds.
5. Serve and enjoy!

Nutritional Information (per serving):
- Calories: 320
- Protein: 8g
- Carbohydrates: 55g
- Fat: 9g
- Fiber: 7g

Spinach and Feta Omelette

- **Total Time:** 15 minutes
- **Servings:** 1

Ingredients:
- 2 large eggs
- 1 cup fresh spinach, chopped
- 1/4 cup feta cheese, crumbled

- Salt and pepper to taste
- 1 teaspoon olive oil

Directions:
1. In a bowl, whisk the eggs and season with salt and pepper.
2. Heat olive oil in a non-stick skillet over medium heat.
3. Add chopped spinach to the skillet and sauté until wilted.
4. Pour whisked eggs over the spinach and let them set slightly.
5. Sprinkle feta cheese over one half of the omelette.
6. Carefully fold the other half over the cheese and cook until eggs are fully set.
7. Slide the omelette onto a plate and serve.

Nutritional Information:
- Calories: 320
- Protein: 20g
- Carbohydrates: 4g
- Fat: 25g
- Fiber: 2g

Blueberry and Greek Yogurt Parfait

- **Total Time:** 10 minutes
- **Servings:** 1

Ingredients:
- 1 cup Greek yogurt
- 1/2 cup blueberries
- 1/4 cup granola
- 1 tablespoon honey
- Fresh mint leaves (optional, for garnish)

Directions:
1. In a glass or bowl, layer Greek yogurt, blueberries, and granola.
2. Drizzle honey over the top.
3. Garnish with fresh mint leaves if desired.
4. Repeat the layering process if making multiple servings.
5. Serve immediately and enjoy!

Nutritional Information:
- Calories: 350
- Protein: 20g

- Carbohydrates: 45g
- Fat: 10g
- Fiber: 6g

Avocado Toast with Poached Egg

- **Total Time:** 15 minutes
- **Servings:** 2

Ingredients:
- 2 slices whole-grain bread, toasted
- 1 ripe avocado, mashed
- 2 large eggs, poached
- Salt and pepper to taste
- Red pepper flakes (optional, for garnish)

Directions:
1. Spread mashed avocado evenly over toasted bread slices.
2. Top each slice with a poached egg.
3. Season with salt, pepper, and red pepper flakes if desired.
4. Serve immediately for a delicious and nutritious breakfast.

Nutritional Information (per serving):
- Calories: 320
- Protein: 14g
- Carbohydrates: 25g
- Fat: 20g
- Fiber: 8g

Chia Seed Pudding with Mango

- **Total Time:** 4 hours (including chilling time)
- **Servings:** 2

Ingredients:
- 1/4 cup chia seeds
- 1 cup almond milk
- 1 tablespoon honey
- 1/2 teaspoon vanilla extract
- 1 ripe mango, diced

Directions:

1. In a bowl, mix chia seeds, almond milk, honey, and vanilla extract.
2. Stir well and refrigerate for at least 4 hours or overnight, allowing the chia seeds to absorb the liquid.
3. Once set, spoon the chia pudding into serving glasses.
4. Top with diced mango.
5. Serve chilled and enjoy this nutrient-packed pudding.

Nutritional Information (per serving):

- Calories: 220
- Protein: 5g
- Carbohydrates: 35g
- Fat: 8g
- Fiber: 10g

Salmon and Cream Cheese Bagel

- **Total Time:** 15 minutes
- **Servings:** 1

Ingredients:

- 1 whole-grain bagel, sliced and toasted
- 2 ounces smoked salmon
- 2 tablespoons cream cheese
- Capers (optional, for garnish)
- Fresh dill (optional, for garnish)
- Lemon wedges (for serving)

Directions:

1. Spread cream cheese on the toasted bagel halves.
2. Top with smoked salmon.
3. Garnish with capers and fresh dill if desired.
4. Serve with lemon wedges on the side.

Nutritional Information:

- Calories: 380
- Protein: 25g
- Carbohydrates: 35g
- Fat: 16g
- Fiber: 5g

Whole Grain Pancakes with Walnuts

- **Total Time:** 25 minutes
- **Servings:** 2 (about 6 pancakes)

Ingredients:
- 1 cup whole wheat flour
- 2 tablespoons ground flaxseed
- 1 tablespoon sugar
- 1 teaspoon baking powder
- 1/2 teaspoon baking soda
- 1 cup buttermilk
- 1 large egg
- 1 tablespoon melted butter
- 1/4 cup chopped walnuts

Directions:
1. In a large bowl, whisk together flour, flaxseed, sugar, baking powder, and baking soda.
2. In a separate bowl, whisk together buttermilk, egg, and melted butter.
3. Pour the wet ingredients into the dry ingredients and stir until just combined.
4. Fold in chopped walnuts.
5. Heat a griddle or non-stick skillet over medium heat.
6. Spoon batter onto the griddle to form pancakes and cook until bubbles form on the surface.
7. Flip the pancakes and cook until golden brown on the other side.
8. Serve warm with your favorite toppings.

Nutritional Information (per serving):
- Calories: 320
- Protein: 11g
- Carbohydrates: 40g
- Fat: 15g
- Fiber: 7g

Vegetable and Tofu Scramble

- **Total Time:** 15 minutes
- **Servings:** 2

Ingredients:
- 1 tablespoon olive oil
- 1/2 cup red bell pepper, diced
- 1/2 cup green bell pepper, diced
- 1/2 cup red onion, diced
- 1 cup firm tofu, crumbled
- 1 teaspoon turmeric
- Salt and pepper to taste
- Fresh herbs (parsley or chives) for garnish

Directions:
1. Heat olive oil in a skillet over medium heat.
2. Add red bell pepper, green bell pepper, and red onion. Sauté until vegetables are tender.
3. Stir in crumbled tofu and sprinkle with turmeric, salt, and pepper.
4. Cook until tofu is heated through.
5. Garnish with fresh herbs and serve.

Nutritional Information (per serving):
- Calories: 180
- Protein: 12g
- Carbohydrates: 10g
- Fat: 11g
- Fiber: 3g

Almond Butter Banana Smoothie Bowl

- **Total Time:** 10 minutes
- **Servings:** 1

Ingredients:
- 1 large banana, frozen
- 1/2 cup almond milk
- 2 tablespoons almond butter
- 1/4 cup granola
- 1 tablespoon chia seeds
- Sliced banana and almonds for topping

Directions:
1. In a blender, combine frozen banana, almond milk, and almond butter.
2. Blend until smooth and creamy.
3. Pour into a bowl and top with granola, chia seeds, sliced banana, and almonds.
4. Serve immediately.

Nutritional Information:
- Calories: 420
- Protein: 10g
- Carbohydrates: 50g
- Fat: 22g
- Fiber: 8g

Sweet Potato Hash with Turkey Sausage

- **Total Time:** 30 minutes
- **Servings:** 2

Ingredients:
- 2 medium sweet potatoes, peeled and diced
- 1/2 pound turkey sausage, crumbled
- 1/2 cup red bell pepper, diced
- 1/2 cup green bell pepper, diced
- 1/2 cup red onion, diced
- 1 teaspoon paprika
- Salt and pepper to taste
- 2 tablespoons olive oil
- Poached eggs (optional, for serving)

Directions:
1. In a large skillet, heat olive oil over medium heat.
2. Add sweet potatoes, turkey sausage, red bell pepper, green bell pepper, and red onion.
3. Cook until sweet potatoes are tender and sausage is browned.
4. Season with paprika, salt, and pepper.
5. Optionally, serve with poached eggs on top.

Nutritional Information (per serving):
- Calories: 380
- Protein: 18g
- Carbohydrates: 30g

- Fat: 20g
- Fiber: 5g

Greek Yogurt and Berry Smoothie

- **Total Time:** 10 minutes
- **Servings:** 1

Ingredients:
- 1 cup Greek yogurt
- 1/2 cup mixed berries (strawberries, blueberries, raspberries)
- 1/2 banana
- 1/2 cup spinach (optional)
- 1 tablespoon honey
- Ice cubes (optional)

Directions:
1. In a blender, combine Greek yogurt, mixed berries, banana, and spinach.
2. Add honey and blend until smooth.
3. If desired, add ice cubes and blend again for a colder consistency.
4. Pour into a glass and enjoy this protein-packed smoothie.

Nutritional Information:
- Calories: 320
- Protein: 25g
- Carbohydrates: 45g
- Fat: 5g
- Fiber: 6g

Oatmeal with Pecans and Dried Cranberries

- **Total Time:** 15 minutes
- **Servings:** 2

Ingredients:
- 1 cup rolled oats
- 2 cups water or milk
- 1/4 cup pecans, chopped
- 1/4 cup dried cranberries
- 1 tablespoon maple syrup
- Pinch of cinnamon
- Fresh berries for topping

Directions:

1. In a saucepan, bring water or milk to a boil.
2. Stir in rolled oats and reduce heat to simmer. Cook until oats are tender.
3. Mix in chopped pecans, dried cranberries, maple syrup, and cinnamon.
4. Continue to cook until the mixture thickens.
5. Serve hot, topped with fresh berries.

Nutritional Information (per serving):

- Calories: 280
- Protein: 7g
- Carbohydrates: 45g
- Fat: 9g
- Fiber: 6g

Breakfast Burrito with Black Beans and Salsa

- **Total Time:** 20 minutes
- **Servings:** 2

Ingredients:

- 4 large eggs, scrambled
- 1 cup black beans, cooked
- 1/2 cup salsa
- 1/4 cup shredded cheddar cheese
- 2 whole wheat tortillas
- Avocado slices for garnish
- Fresh cilantro for garnish

Directions:

1. In a skillet, scramble the eggs until cooked through.
2. Warm the black beans and tortillas.
3. Assemble each burrito with scrambled eggs, black beans, salsa, and shredded cheddar.
4. Garnish with avocado slices and fresh cilantro.
5. Fold the tortillas and serve.

Nutritional Information (per serving):

- Calories: 380
- Protein: 20g
- Carbohydrates: 40g
- Fat: 15g
- Fiber: 10g

Cottage Cheese and Pineapple Bowl

- **Total Time:** 5 minutes
- **Servings:** 1

Ingredients:
- 1 cup cottage cheese
- 1 cup fresh pineapple chunks
- 1 tablespoon honey
- 2 tablespoons chopped walnuts

Directions:
1. In a bowl, combine cottage cheese and fresh pineapple chunks.
2. Drizzle with honey and sprinkle chopped walnuts on top.
3. Stir gently to combine.
4. Serve immediately for a quick and satisfying breakfast.

Nutritional Information:
- Calories: 320
- Protein: 25g
- Carbohydrates: 35g
- Fat: 12g
- Fiber: 3g

Whole Wheat English Muffin with Smoked Salmon

- **Total Time:** 10 minutes
- **Servings:** 1

Ingredients:
- 1 whole wheat English muffin, toasted
- 2 ounces smoked salmon
- 2 tablespoons cream cheese
- Capers for garnish
- Fresh dill for garnish
- Lemon wedges for serving

Directions:
1. Spread cream cheese on the toasted English muffin.
2. Top with smoked salmon.
3. Garnish with capers and fresh dill.

4. Serve with lemon wedges on the side.

Nutritional Information:
- Calories: 280
- Protein: 20g
- Carbohydrates: 25g
- Fat: 12g
- Fiber: 5g

Lunch

Lentil and Vegetable Soup

- **Total Time:** 45 minutes
- **Servings:** 4

Ingredients:
- 1 cup dried green lentils, rinsed
- 1 onion, diced
- 2 carrots, diced
- 2 celery stalks, diced
- 3 cloves garlic, minced
- 1 can (14 oz) diced tomatoes
- 4 cups vegetable broth
- 1 teaspoon ground cumin
- 1 teaspoon smoked paprika
- Salt and pepper to taste
- Fresh parsley for garnish

Directions:
1. In a large pot, sauté onion, carrots, and celery until softened.
2. Add garlic and cook for another minute.
3. Stir in lentils, diced tomatoes, vegetable broth, cumin, and smoked paprika.
4. Bring to a boil, then reduce heat and simmer for 30-35 minutes or until lentils are tender.
5. Season with salt and pepper to taste.
6. Garnish with fresh parsley and serve.

Nutritional Information (per serving):
- Calories: 250
- Protein: 15g
- Carbohydrates: 45g
- Fat: 1g
- Fiber: 15g

Quinoa Salad with Grilled Chicken

- **Total Time:** 30 minutes
- **Servings:** 3

Ingredients:
- 1 cup quinoa, cooked
- 1 grilled chicken breast, sliced
- 1 cup cherry tomatoes, halved
- 1 cucumber, diced
- 1/4 cup red onion, finely chopped
- Feta cheese, crumbled (optional)
- Fresh basil, chopped
- Balsamic vinaigrette dressing

Directions:
1. In a bowl, combine cooked quinoa, grilled chicken, cherry tomatoes, cucumber, and red onion.
2. If desired, sprinkle with crumbled feta cheese.
3. Drizzle with balsamic vinaigrette dressing and toss to combine.
4. Garnish with fresh basil.
5. Serve chilled or at room temperature.

Nutritional Information (per serving):
- Calories: 380
- Protein: 30g
- Carbohydrates: 40g
- Fat: 12g
- Fiber: 7g

Turkey and Avocado Wrap

- **Total Time:** 15 minutes
- **Servings:** 2

Ingredients:
- 8 oz deli turkey slices
- 2 whole wheat wraps
- 1 avocado, sliced
- 1 cup mixed greens
- 1/4 cup cherry tomatoes, halved
- 2 tablespoons Greek yogurt dressing

Directions:

1. Lay out the whole wheat wraps and layer with turkey slices.
2. Top with avocado slices, mixed greens, and cherry tomatoes.
3. Drizzle with Greek yogurt dressing.
4. Roll up the wraps, slice in half, and serve.

Nutritional Information (per serving):

- Calories: 380
- Protein: 25g
- Carbohydrates: 30g
- Fat: 18g
- Fiber: 8g

Chickpea and Spinach Stew

- **Total Time:** 40 minutes
- **Servings:** 4

Ingredients:

- 2 tablespoons olive oil
- 1 onion, diced
- 3 cloves garlic, minced
- 1 teaspoon ground cumin
- 1 teaspoon ground coriander
- 1 teaspoon smoked paprika
- 2 cans (15 oz each) chickpeas, drained and rinsed
- 1 can (14 oz) diced tomatoes
- 4 cups vegetable broth
- 4 cups fresh spinach
- Salt and pepper to taste
- Lemon wedges for serving

Directions:

1. In a large pot, heat olive oil and sauté onion and garlic until softened.
2. Add ground cumin, coriander, and smoked paprika. Cook for another minute.
3. Stir in chickpeas, diced tomatoes, and vegetable broth.
4. Bring to a simmer and cook for 20 minutes.
5. Add fresh spinach and cook until wilted.
6. Season with salt and pepper to taste.
7. Serve with a squeeze of lemon.

Nutritional Information (per serving):
- Calories: 280
- Protein: 15g
- Carbohydrates: 45g
- Fat: 7g
- Fiber: 12g

Tuna Salad Lettuce Wraps

- **Total Time:** 15 minutes
- **Servings:** 2

Ingredients:
- 1 can (5 oz) tuna, drained
- 1/4 cup red onion, finely chopped
- 1/4 cup celery, finely chopped
- 2 tablespoons mayonnaise
- 1 tablespoon Dijon mustard
- Salt and pepper to taste
- Butter lettuce leaves

Directions:
1. In a bowl, mix tuna, red onion, celery, mayonnaise, and Dijon mustard.
2. Season with salt and pepper to taste.
3. Spoon tuna salad onto butter lettuce leaves.
4. Wrap and secure with toothpicks if needed.
5. Serve as a light and refreshing lunch.

Nutritional Information (per serving):
- Calories: 220
- Protein: 20g
- Carbohydrates: 5g
- Fat: 14g
- Fiber: 2g

Roasted Vegetable and Hummus Wrap

- **Total Time:** 25 minutes
- **Servings:** 2

Ingredients:
- 2 whole wheat wraps
- 1 cup mixed vegetables (bell peppers, zucchini, eggplant), sliced
- 2 tablespoons olive oil
- Salt and pepper to taste
- 1/2 cup hummus
- Fresh parsley, chopped
- Lemon wedges for serving

Directions:
1. Preheat the oven to 400°F (200°C).
2. Toss mixed vegetables with olive oil, salt, and pepper.
3. Roast in the oven for 20 minutes or until vegetables are tender.
4. Spread hummus on whole wheat wraps.
5. Top with roasted vegetables and sprinkle with fresh parsley.
6. Roll up the wraps and serve with lemon wedges.

Nutritional Information (per serving):
- Calories: 320
- Protein: 10g
- Carbohydrates: 40g
- Fat: 15g
- Fiber: 8g

Brown Rice Bowl with Teriyaki Salmon

- **Total Time:** 30 minutes
- **Servings:** 2

Ingredients:
- 1 cup brown rice, cooked
- 2 salmon fillets
- 1/4 cup teriyaki sauce
- 1 cup broccoli florets
- 1 carrot, julienned
- 1/4 cup green onions, chopped
- Sesame seeds for garnish

Directions:

1. Marinate salmon fillets in teriyaki sauce for 15 minutes.
2. In a skillet, cook salmon until browned on both sides and cooked through.
3. Steam broccoli until tender-crisp.
4. Assemble bowls with brown rice, teriyaki salmon, steamed broccoli, julienned carrot, and chopped green onions.
5. Garnish with sesame seeds.
6. Serve immediately.

Nutritional Information (per serving):

- Calories: 400
- Protein: 25g
- Carbohydrates: 45g
- Fat: 15g
- Fiber: 6g

Grilled Portobello Mushroom Salad

- **Total Time:** 25 minutes
- **Servings:** 2

Ingredients:

- 4 large portobello mushrooms, cleaned and stems removed
- 2 tablespoons balsamic vinegar
- 3 tablespoons olive oil
- 2 cloves garlic, minced
- Salt and pepper to taste
- Mixed salad greens
- Cherry tomatoes, halved
- Red onion, thinly sliced
- Feta cheese, crumbled
- Balsamic vinaigrette dressing

Directions:

1. In a bowl, whisk together balsamic vinegar, olive oil, minced garlic, salt, and pepper.
2. Brush the portobello mushrooms with the dressing and grill until tender.
3. Slice the grilled mushrooms and arrange them on a bed of mixed salad greens.
4. Add cherry tomatoes, red onion, and crumbled feta.
5. Drizzle with balsamic vinaigrette dressing.
6. Serve and enjoy this flavorful mushroom salad.

Nutritional Information (per serving):
- Calories: 280
- Protein: 12g
- Carbohydrates: 20g
- Fat: 20g
- Fiber: 6g

Whole Wheat Pita with Greek Salad

- **Total Time:** 15 minutes
- **Servings:** 2

Ingredients:
- 2 whole wheat pitas, cut in half
- 1 cucumber, diced
- 1 cup cherry tomatoes, halved
- 1/2 cup Kalamata olives, sliced
- 1/2 cup feta cheese, crumbled
- Red onion, thinly sliced
- Fresh parsley, chopped
- Greek dressing

Directions:
1. In a bowl, combine diced cucumber, cherry tomatoes, Kalamata olives, crumbled feta, red onion, and chopped fresh parsley.
2. Toss the salad with Greek dressing.
3. Warm the whole wheat pitas.
4. Stuff each pita half with the Greek salad mixture.
5. Serve these delicious and portable Greek salad pockets.

Nutritional Information (per serving):
- Calories: 320
- Protein: 10g
- Carbohydrates: 45g
- Fat: 12g
- Fiber: 8g

Broccoli and Cheddar Stuffed Baked Potatoes

- **Total Time:** 1 hour
- **Servings:** 4

Ingredients:
- 4 large baking potatoes
- 2 cups broccoli florets, steamed
- 1 cup sharp cheddar cheese, shredded
- 1/2 cup plain Greek yogurt
- Salt and pepper to taste
- Chives, chopped (for garnish)

Directions:
1. Preheat the oven to 400°F (200°C).
2. Pierce each potato with a fork and bake for 45-50 minutes or until tender.
3. Cut a slit in each potato and fluff the insides with a fork.
4. In a bowl, mix steamed broccoli, shredded cheddar, Greek yogurt, salt, and pepper.
5. Stuff each potato with the broccoli and cheddar mixture.
6. Garnish with chopped chives.
7. Serve these hearty stuffed baked potatoes.

Nutritional Information (per serving):
- Calories: 320
- Protein: 15g
- Carbohydrates: 50g
- Fat: 8g
- Fiber: 7g

Quinoa and Black Bean Burrito Bowl

- **Total Time:** 30 minutes
- **Servings:** 2

Ingredients:
- 1 cup quinoa, cooked
- 1 can (15 oz) black beans, drained and rinsed
- 1 cup corn kernels (fresh or frozen)
- 1 cup cherry tomatoes, halved
- 1 avocado, sliced

- Fresh cilantro, chopped
- Lime wedges
- Salsa (optional)

Directions:
1. In a bowl, assemble cooked quinoa, black beans, corn, cherry tomatoes, and sliced avocado.
2. Garnish with chopped cilantro.
3. Serve with lime wedges and salsa on the side.
4. Enjoy this wholesome and customizable burrito bowl.

Nutritional Information (per serving):
- Calories: 380
- Protein: 15g
- Carbohydrates: 60g
- Fat: 12g
- Fiber: 12g

Mediterranean Chicken Salad

- **Total Time:** 20 minutes
- **Servings:** 3

Ingredients:
- 1 pound chicken breast, grilled and sliced
- 2 cups mixed salad greens
- 1 cup cherry tomatoes, halved
- 1 cucumber, diced
- 1/2 cup Kalamata olives, sliced
- 1/4 cup red onion, thinly sliced
- Feta cheese, crumbled
- Greek dressing

Directions:
1. In a large salad bowl, combine grilled chicken slices, mixed salad greens, cherry tomatoes, diced cucumber, sliced Kalamata olives, and thinly sliced red onion.
2. Toss the salad with crumbled feta and Greek dressing.
3. Serve this refreshing and protein-packed Mediterranean chicken salad.

Nutritional Information (per serving):
- Calories: 320

- Protein: 30g
- Carbohydrates: 15g
- Fat: 18g
- Fiber: 5g

Barley and Vegetable Stir-Fry

- **Total Time:** 25 minutes
- **Servings:** 4

Ingredients:
- 1 cup pearl barley, cooked
- 2 tablespoons soy sauce
- 1 tablespoon sesame oil
- 1 tablespoon hoisin sauce
- 1 tablespoon rice vinegar
- 2 tablespoons vegetable oil
- 1 cup broccoli florets
- 1 bell pepper, thinly sliced
- 1 carrot, julienned
- 2 cloves garlic, minced
- Green onions, chopped (for garnish)
- Sesame seeds (for garnish)

Directions:
1. In a bowl, whisk together soy sauce, sesame oil, hoisin sauce, and rice vinegar.
2. Heat vegetable oil in a wok or skillet.
3. Stir-fry broccoli, bell pepper, carrot, and minced garlic until vegetables are tender-crisp.
4. Add cooked barley and pour the sauce over the stir-fry.
5. Toss everything together until well combined.
6. Garnish with chopped green onions and sesame seeds.
7. Serve this flavorful barley and vegetable stir-fry.

Nutritional Information (per serving):
- Calories: 280
- Protein: 8g
- Carbohydrates: 45g
- Fat: 10g
- Fiber: 8g

Shrimp and Quinoa Spring Rolls

- **Total Time:** 30 minutes
- **Servings:** 2

Ingredients:
- 1 cup quinoa, cooked
- 10 rice paper wrappers
- 1/2 pound cooked shrimp, peeled and deveined
- 1 cup cucumber, julienned
- 1 cup carrots, julienned
- Fresh mint leaves
- Fresh cilantro leaves
- Peanut dipping sauce

Directions:
1. Dip a rice paper wrapper into warm water until pliable.
2. Lay the wrapper flat and add a small portion of cooked quinoa, shrimp, cucumber, carrots, mint, and cilantro.
3. Fold in the sides of the wrapper and roll tightly.
4. Repeat with remaining ingredients.
5. Serve these shrimp and quinoa spring rolls with peanut dipping sauce.

Nutritional Information (per serving):
- Calories: 320
- Protein: 20g
- Carbohydrates: 50g
- Fat: 5g
- Fiber: 6g

Caprese Sandwich with Whole Grain Bread

- **Total Time:** 15 minutes
- **Servings:** 2

Ingredients:
- 4 slices whole grain bread
- 2 large tomatoes, sliced
- 8 ounces fresh mozzarella, sliced
- Fresh basil leaves
- Balsamic glaze

- Olive oil
- Salt and pepper to taste

Directions:
1. Toast the whole grain bread slices.
2. Layer each slice with tomato, fresh mozzarella, and basil leaves.
3. Drizzle with balsamic glaze and olive oil.
4. Season with salt and pepper to taste.
5. Assemble the slices to create delicious caprese sandwiches.

Nutritional Information (per serving):
- Calories: 380
- Protein: 18g
- Carbohydrates: 30g
- Fat: 20g
- Fiber: 5g

Dinner

Baked Lemon Herb Salmon

- **Total Time:** 25 minutes
- **Servings:** 2

Ingredients:
- 2 salmon fillets
- 2 tablespoons olive oil
- 1 lemon, juiced
- 2 cloves garlic, minced
- 1 teaspoon dried thyme
- 1 teaspoon dried rosemary
- Salt and pepper to taste
- Fresh parsley for garnish

Directions:
1. Preheat the oven to 400°F (200°C).
2. Place salmon fillets on a baking sheet lined with parchment paper.
3. In a bowl, mix together olive oil, lemon juice, minced garlic, dried thyme, dried rosemary, salt, and pepper.
4. Pour the mixture over the salmon fillets.
5. Bake for 15-20 minutes or until the salmon is cooked through.
6. Garnish with fresh parsley before serving.

Nutritional Information (per serving):
- Calories: 320
- Protein: 30g
- Carbohydrates: 2g
- Fat: 22g
- Fiber: 1g

Spaghetti Squash with Turkey Bolognese

- **Total Time:** 45 minutes
- **Servings:** 4

Ingredients:
- 1 large spaghetti squash

- 1 pound ground turkey
- 1 onion, diced
- 2 cloves garlic, minced
- 1 can (14 oz) crushed tomatoes
- 1 teaspoon dried oregano
- 1 teaspoon dried basil
- Salt and pepper to taste
- Parmesan cheese for garnish
- Fresh basil for garnish

Directions:
1. Preheat the oven to 400°F (200°C).
2. Cut the spaghetti squash in half lengthwise and scoop out the seeds.
3. Place the squash halves on a baking sheet, cut side down, and roast for 30-40 minutes or until tender.
4. In a skillet, cook ground turkey, onion, and garlic until turkey is browned.
5. Stir in crushed tomatoes, dried oregano, dried basil, salt, and pepper.
6. Use a fork to scrape the cooked spaghetti squash into strands.
7. Serve the turkey Bolognese over spaghetti squash.
8. Garnish with Parmesan cheese and fresh basil.

Nutritional Information (per serving):
- Calories: 280
- Protein: 25g
- Carbohydrates: 20g
- Fat: 12g
- Fiber: 5g

Grilled Vegetable and Chicken Kebabs

- **Total Time:** 30 minutes
- **Servings:** 4

Ingredients:
- 1 pound boneless, skinless chicken breast, cut into cubes
- 1 zucchini, sliced
- 1 red bell pepper, diced
- 1 yellow bell pepper, diced
- 1 red onion, diced
- Cherry tomatoes
- 2 tablespoons olive oil

- 1 teaspoon dried oregano
- 1 teaspoon dried thyme
- Salt and pepper to taste
- Lemon wedges for serving

Directions:
1. Preheat the grill to medium-high heat.
2. In a bowl, combine chicken cubes, zucchini, red bell pepper, yellow bell pepper, red onion, and cherry tomatoes.
3. Drizzle with olive oil and sprinkle with dried oregano, dried thyme, salt, and pepper. Toss to coat.
4. Thread the chicken and vegetables onto skewers.
5. Grill kebabs for 12-15 minutes, turning occasionally, until chicken is cooked through.
6. Serve with lemon wedges.

Nutritional Information (per serving):
- Calories: 280
- Protein: 30g
- Carbohydrates: 10g
- Fat: 12g
- Fiber: 3g

Quinoa-Stuffed Bell Peppers

- **Total Time:** 50 minutes
- **Servings:** 4

Ingredients:
- 4 large bell peppers, halved and seeds removed
- 1 cup quinoa, cooked
- 1 pound lean ground beef or turkey
- 1 onion, diced
- 2 cloves garlic, minced
- 1 can (14 oz) diced tomatoes
- 1 teaspoon cumin
- 1 teaspoon chili powder
- Salt and pepper to taste
- Shredded cheddar cheese for topping
- Fresh cilantro for garnish

Directions:

1. Preheat the oven to 375°F (190°C).
2. Place bell pepper halves in a baking dish.
3. In a skillet, cook ground beef or turkey, onion, and garlic until meat is browned.
4. Stir in cooked quinoa, diced tomatoes, cumin, chili powder, salt, and pepper.
5. Spoon the quinoa mixture into bell pepper halves.
6. Top with shredded cheddar cheese.
7. Bake for 25-30 minutes or until peppers are tender.
8. Garnish with fresh cilantro before serving.

Nutritional Information (per serving):

- Calories: 350
- Protein: 25g
- Carbohydrates: 30g
- Fat: 15g
- Fiber: 6g

Sweet and Spicy Grilled Shrimp

- **Total Time:** 20 minutes
- **Servings:** 2

Ingredients:

- 1 pound large shrimp, peeled and deveined
- 2 tablespoons olive oil
- 2 tablespoons honey
- 1 tablespoon soy sauce
- 1 teaspoon chili powder
- 1 teaspoon garlic powder
- 1/2 teaspoon cayenne pepper (adjust to taste)
- Lemon wedges for serving

Directions:

1. Preheat the grill to medium-high heat.
2. In a bowl, whisk together olive oil, honey, soy sauce, chili powder, garlic powder, and cayenne pepper.
3. Toss shrimp in the marinade until well coated.
4. Thread shrimp on skewers.
5. Grill shrimp for 2-3 minutes per side or until opaque and lightly charred.
6. Serve with lemon wedges.

Nutritional Information (per serving):
- Calories: 280
- Protein: 25g
- Carbohydrates: 15g
- Fat: 14g
- Fiber: 1g

Turkey and Vegetable Stir-Fry

- **Total Time:** 25 minutes
- **Servings:** 4

Ingredients:
- 1 pound ground turkey
- 2 tablespoons soy sauce
- 1 tablespoon hoisin sauce
- 1 tablespoon sesame oil
- 1 tablespoon vegetable oil
- 1 bell pepper, thinly sliced
- 1 zucchini, sliced
- 1 carrot, julienned
- 2 cups broccoli florets
- 2 cloves garlic, minced
- 1 teaspoon ginger, grated
- Green onions, chopped (for garnish)
- Sesame seeds (for garnish)
- Brown rice or quinoa (for serving)

Directions:
1. In a bowl, mix ground turkey with soy sauce, hoisin sauce, and sesame oil.
2. Heat vegetable oil in a wok or skillet.
3. Add ground turkey mixture and cook until browned.
4. Add bell pepper, zucchini, carrot, broccoli, garlic, and ginger. Stir-fry until vegetables are tender-crisp.
5. Garnish with chopped green onions and sesame seeds.
6. Serve over brown rice or quinoa.

Nutritional Information (per serving):
- Calories: 320
- Protein: 25g
- Carbohydrates: 20g

- Fat: 15g
- Fiber: 5g

Baked Cod with Garlic and Herbs

- **Total Time:** 20 minutes
- **Servings:** 2

Ingredients:
- 2 cod fillets
- 2 tablespoons olive oil
- 3 cloves garlic, minced
- 1 tablespoon fresh parsley, chopped
- 1 teaspoon dried thyme
- Salt and pepper to taste
- Lemon wedges for serving

Directions:
1. Preheat the oven to 400°F (200°C).
2. Place cod fillets on a baking sheet lined with parchment paper.
3. In a bowl, mix together olive oil, minced garlic, chopped fresh parsley, dried thyme, salt, and pepper.
4. Spread the mixture over the cod fillets.
5. Bake for 12-15 minutes or until the cod is opaque and flakes easily.
6. Serve with lemon wedges.

Nutritional Information (per serving):
- Calories: 280
- Protein: 30g
- Carbohydrates: 2g
- Fat: 18g
- Fiber: 1g

Eggplant and Chickpea Curry

- **Total Time:** 40 minutes
- **Servings:** 4

Ingredients:
- 1 large eggplant, cubed
- 1 can (15 oz) chickpeas, drained and rinsed

- 1 onion, diced
- 2 cloves garlic, minced
- 1 can (14 oz) diced tomatoes
- 1 can (14 oz) coconut milk
- 2 tablespoons curry powder
- 1 teaspoon ground cumin
- 1 teaspoon ground coriander
- Salt and pepper to taste
- Fresh cilantro for garnish
- Cooked basmati rice (for serving)

Directions:
1. In a large pot, sauté onion and garlic until softened.
2. Add eggplant and cook for 5 minutes.
3. Stir in chickpeas, diced tomatoes, coconut milk, curry powder, cumin, coriander, salt, and pepper.
4. Simmer for 20-25 minutes or until the eggplant is tender.
5. Garnish with fresh cilantro and serve over cooked basmati rice.

Nutritional Information (per serving):
- Calories: 320
- Protein: 10g
- Carbohydrates: 40g
- Fat: 15g
- Fiber: 12g

Grilled Tofu and Vegetable Skewers

- **Total Time:** 30 minutes
- **Servings:** 3

Ingredients:
- 1 block extra-firm tofu, pressed and cubed
- 1 zucchini, sliced
- 1 bell pepper, diced
- 1 red onion, diced
- Cherry tomatoes
- 2 tablespoons olive oil
- 1 teaspoon smoked paprika
- 1 teaspoon cumin
- Salt and pepper to taste
- Lemon wedges for serving

Directions:

1. Preheat the grill to medium-high heat.
2. In a bowl, toss cubed tofu, zucchini, bell pepper, red onion, and cherry tomatoes with olive oil, smoked paprika, cumin, salt, and pepper.
3. Thread the tofu and vegetables onto skewers.
4. Grill for 10-12 minutes, turning occasionally, until the tofu is golden and the vegetables are tender.
5. Serve with lemon wedges.

Nutritional Information (per serving):

- Calories: 280
- Protein: 15g
- Carbohydrates: 15g
- Fat: 18g
- Fiber: 5g

Spinach and Mushroom Stuffed Chicken Breast

- **Total Time:** 35 minutes
- **Servings:** 2

Ingredients:

- 2 boneless, skinless chicken breasts
- 1 cup fresh spinach, chopped
- 1/2 cup mushrooms, finely chopped
- 1/4 cup feta cheese, crumbled
- 2 cloves garlic, minced
- Salt and pepper to taste
- Olive oil for cooking

Directions:

1. Preheat the oven to 375°F (190°C).
2. In a bowl, mix chopped spinach, mushrooms, feta cheese, minced garlic, salt, and pepper.
3. Cut a pocket into each chicken breast.
4. Stuff the chicken breasts with the spinach and mushroom mixture.
5. Heat olive oil in an oven-safe skillet.
6. Sear the chicken breasts for 2-3 minutes on each side.
7. Transfer the skillet to the oven and bake for 20-25 minutes or until the chicken is cooked through.

Nutritional Information (per serving):
- Calories: 320
- Protein: 40g
- Carbohydrates: 5g
- Fat: 16g
- Fiber: 2g

Cauliflower and Lentil Curry

- **Total Time:** 45 minutes
- **Servings:** 4

Ingredients:
- 1 head cauliflower, cut into florets
- 1 cup dry lentils, rinsed
- 1 onion, diced
- 2 cloves garlic, minced
- 1 can (14 oz) diced tomatoes
- 1 can (14 oz) coconut milk
- 2 tablespoons curry powder
- 1 teaspoon ground turmeric
- 1 teaspoon ground cumin
- Salt and pepper to taste
- Fresh cilantro for garnish
- Cooked brown rice (for serving)

Directions:
1. In a large pot, sauté onion and garlic until softened.
2. Add cauliflower, lentils, diced tomatoes, coconut milk, curry powder, turmeric, cumin, salt, and pepper.
3. Simmer for 30-35 minutes or until the lentils are tender.
4. Garnish with fresh cilantro and serve over cooked brown rice.

Nutritional Information (per serving):
- Calories: 380
- Protein: 20g
- Carbohydrates: 50g
- Fat: 15g
- Fiber: 15g

Lemon Garlic Herb Grilled Chicken

- **Total Time:** 25 minutes
- **Servings:** 2

Ingredients:
- 2 boneless, skinless chicken breasts
- 2 tablespoons olive oil
- 2 cloves garlic, minced
- Zest and juice of 1 lemon
- 1 teaspoon dried thyme
- 1 teaspoon dried rosemary
- Salt and pepper to taste

Directions:
1. In a bowl, mix olive oil, minced garlic, lemon zest, lemon juice, dried thyme, dried rosemary, salt, and pepper.
2. Marinate the chicken breasts in the mixture for at least 15 minutes.
3. Preheat the grill to medium-high heat.
4. Grill the chicken for 6-8 minutes per side or until cooked through.
5. Let the chicken rest for a few minutes before serving.

Nutritional Information (per serving):
- Calories: 280
- Protein: 30g
- Carbohydrates: 2g
- Fat: 18g
- Fiber: 1g

Whole Wheat Pasta with Tomato and Basil

- **Total Time:** 20 minutes
- **Servings:** 3

Ingredients:
- 8 oz whole wheat pasta
- 2 tablespoons olive oil
- 3 cloves garlic, minced
- 1 can (14 oz) diced tomatoes
- Fresh basil, chopped
- Red pepper flakes (optional)

- Salt and pepper to taste
- Grated Parmesan cheese for topping

Directions:

1. Cook the whole wheat pasta according to package instructions.
2. In a skillet, sauté minced garlic in olive oil until fragrant.
3. Add diced tomatoes and cook for 5 minutes.
4. Toss the cooked pasta with the tomato mixture.
5. Stir in fresh basil and red pepper flakes if desired.
6. Season with salt and pepper.
7. Top with grated Parmesan cheese before serving.

Nutritional Information (per serving):

- Calories: 320
- Protein: 10g
- Carbohydrates: 50g
- Fat: 10g
- Fiber: 8g

Zucchini Noodles with Pesto and Cherry Tomatoes

- **Total Time:** 15 minutes
- **Servings:** 2

Ingredients:

- 2 large zucchini, spiralized
- 1 cup cherry tomatoes, halved
- 1/2 cup basil pesto
- Pine nuts for garnish (optional)
- Grated Parmesan cheese for topping

Directions:

1. Spiralize the zucchini into noodles.
2. In a bowl, toss zucchini noodles with cherry tomatoes and basil pesto.
3. Warm the mixture in a skillet for 3-5 minutes, or until heated through.
4. Garnish with pine nuts if desired and top with grated Parmesan cheese before serving.

Nutritional Information (per serving):

- Calories: 280
- Protein: 8g

- Carbohydrates: 15g
- Fat: 20g
- Fiber: 5g

Beef and Vegetable Lettuce Wraps

- **Total Time:** 30 minutes
- **Servings:** 4

Ingredients:
- 1 pound lean ground beef
- 1 onion, diced
- 2 cloves garlic, minced
- 1 cup mushrooms, finely chopped
- 1 carrot, grated
- 1/4 cup hoisin sauce
- 2 tablespoons soy sauce
- 1 tablespoon sesame oil
- 1 teaspoon fresh ginger, grated
- Bibb or iceberg lettuce leaves (for wrapping)
- Green onions, chopped (for garnish)
- Sesame seeds (for garnish)

Directions:
1. In a skillet, cook ground beef, onion, and garlic until beef is browned.
2. Add mushrooms, grated carrot, hoisin sauce, soy sauce, sesame oil, and grated ginger. Cook for an additional 5 minutes.
3. Spoon the beef and vegetable mixture into lettuce leaves.
4. Garnish with chopped green onions and sesame seeds.
5. Serve these flavorful beef and vegetable lettuce wraps.

Nutritional Information (per serving):
- Calories: 320
- Protein: 25g
- Carbohydrates: 15g
- Fat: 18g
- Fiber: 4g

Grains and Legumes

Quinoa Pilaf with Mixed Vegetables

- **Total Time:** 25 minutes
- **Servings:** 4

Ingredients:
- 1 cup quinoa, rinsed
- 2 cups vegetable broth
- 1 tablespoon olive oil
- 1 onion, diced
- 2 carrots, diced
- 1 bell pepper, diced
- 1 zucchini, diced
- 1 cup frozen peas
- 1/4 cup fresh parsley, chopped
- Salt and pepper to taste
- Lemon wedges for serving

Directions:
1. In a saucepan, bring vegetable broth to a boil.
2. Add quinoa, reduce heat, cover, and simmer for 15 minutes or until quinoa is cooked.
3. In a large skillet, heat olive oil and sauté onion, carrots, bell pepper, and zucchini until tender.
4. Stir in cooked quinoa and frozen peas.
5. Cook for an additional 5 minutes, stirring occasionally.
6. Season with salt and pepper.
7. Garnish with fresh parsley and serve with lemon wedges.

Nutritional Information (per serving):
- Calories: 280
- Protein: 8g
- Carbohydrates: 45g
- Fat: 8g
- Fiber: 7g

Brown Rice and Black Bean Bowl

- **Total Time:** 30 minutes
- **Servings:** 3

Ingredients:
- 1 cup brown rice, cooked
- 1 can (15 oz) black beans, drained and rinsed
- 1 cup corn kernels (fresh or frozen)
- 1 avocado, sliced
- 1/2 cup salsa
- Fresh cilantro, chopped
- Lime wedges for serving

Directions:
1. In a bowl, assemble cooked brown rice, black beans, corn, sliced avocado, and salsa.
2. Toss the ingredients together.
3. Garnish with fresh cilantro.
4. Serve with lime wedges on the side.

Nutritional Information (per serving):
- Calories: 320
- Protein: 10g
- Carbohydrates: 60g
- Fat: 8g
- Fiber: 12g

Barley Risotto with Roasted Butternut Squash

- **Total Time:** 50 minutes
- **Servings:** 4

Ingredients:
- 1 cup pearl barley, rinsed
- 2 tablespoons olive oil
- 1 onion, diced
- 3 cups butternut squash, peeled and diced
- 2 cloves garlic, minced
- 4 cups vegetable broth
- 1/2 cup Parmesan cheese, grated

- Salt and pepper to taste
- Fresh sage leaves for garnish

Directions:
1. In a large pot, heat olive oil and sauté onion until softened.
2. Add diced butternut squash and cook for 10 minutes or until golden.
3. Stir in minced garlic and cook for an additional 2 minutes.
4. Add pearl barley and cook for 2 minutes, stirring constantly.
5. Pour in vegetable broth, bring to a simmer, and cover.
6. Simmer for 30-35 minutes or until barley is tender.
7. Stir in grated Parmesan cheese and season with salt and pepper.
8. Garnish with fresh sage leaves before serving.

Nutritional Information (per serving):
- Calories: 340
- Protein: 10g
- Carbohydrates: 60g
- Fat: 8g
- Fiber: 10g

Lentil and Sweet Potato Curry

- **Total Time:** 40 minutes
- **Servings:** 4

Ingredients:
- 1 cup dry lentils, rinsed
- 2 sweet potatoes, peeled and diced
- 1 onion, diced
- 2 cloves garlic, minced
- 1 can (14 oz) diced tomatoes
- 1 can (14 oz) coconut milk
- 2 tablespoons curry powder
- 1 teaspoon ground turmeric
- 1 teaspoon ground cumin
- Salt and pepper to taste
- Fresh cilantro for garnish
- Cooked basmati rice (for serving)

Directions:

1. In a large pot, combine lentils, sweet potatoes, onion, garlic, diced tomatoes, coconut milk, curry powder, turmeric, cumin, salt, and pepper.
2. Bring to a boil, then reduce heat, cover, and simmer for 25-30 minutes or until lentils and sweet potatoes are tender.
3. Stir occasionally to prevent sticking.
4. Garnish with fresh cilantro and serve over cooked basmati rice.

Nutritional Information (per serving):

- Calories: 380
- Protein: 15g
- Carbohydrates: 50g
- Fat: 15g
- Fiber: 15g

Farro Salad with Roasted Vegetables

- **Total Time:** 35 minutes
- **Servings:** 3

Ingredients:

- 1 cup farro, cooked
- 1 cup cherry tomatoes, halved
- 1 cup asparagus, chopped
- 1 cup bell peppers, diced
- 1/4 cup feta cheese, crumbled
- 2 tablespoons balsamic vinaigrette dressing
- Fresh basil, chopped (for garnish)

Directions:

1. Preheat the oven to 400°F (200°C).
2. On a baking sheet, roast cherry tomatoes, asparagus, and bell peppers for 15-20 minutes or until vegetables are tender.
3. In a bowl, combine cooked farro, roasted vegetables, crumbled feta, and balsamic vinaigrette dressing.
4. Toss the ingredients until well coated.
5. Garnish with fresh chopped basil before serving.

Nutritional Information (per serving):

- Calories: 320
- Protein: 10g

- Carbohydrates: 50g
- Fat: 8g
- Fiber: 10g

Black Bean and Corn Quesadillas

- **Total Time:** 20 minutes
- **Servings:** 3

Ingredients:

- 1 can (15 oz) black beans, drained and rinsed
- 1 cup corn kernels (fresh or frozen)
- 1 bell pepper, diced
- 1/2 red onion, diced
- 1 teaspoon ground cumin
- 1 teaspoon chili powder
- Salt and pepper to taste
- 6 whole wheat tortillas
- 1 cup shredded cheddar cheese
- Olive oil for cooking

Directions:

1. In a bowl, combine black beans, corn, bell pepper, red onion, ground cumin, chili powder, salt, and pepper.
2. Place a tortilla on a flat surface and spoon the black bean mixture onto one half.
3. Sprinkle it with shredded cheddar cheese and fold the tortilla in half.
4. Repeat for the remaining tortillas.
5. Heat olive oil in a skillet and cook quesadillas until golden on both sides.
6. Slice and serve with your favorite salsa or guacamole.

Nutritional Information (per serving):

- Calories: 380
- Protein: 15g
- Carbohydrates: 50g
- Fat: 15g
- Fiber: 10g

Chickpea and Spinach Stuffed Bell Peppers

- **Total Time:** 40 minutes
- **Servings:** 4

Ingredients:
- 4 bell peppers, halved and seeds removed
- 1 can (15 oz) chickpeas, drained and rinsed
- 2 cups baby spinach, chopped
- 1 cup quinoa, cooked
- 1 onion, diced
- 2 cloves garlic, minced
- 1 teaspoon ground cumin
- 1 teaspoon paprika
- Salt and pepper to taste
- 1 cup tomato sauce
- Feta cheese for topping (optional)

Directions:
1. Preheat the oven to 375°F (190°C).
2. In a skillet, sauté onion and garlic until softened.
3. Add chickpeas, chopped spinach, cooked quinoa, ground cumin, paprika, salt, and pepper. Cook for 5 minutes.
4. Spoon the chickpea mixture into bell pepper halves.
5. Pour tomato sauce over the stuffed peppers.
6. Bake for 25-30 minutes or until peppers are tender.
7. Optional: Top with crumbled feta cheese before serving.

Nutritional Information (per serving):
- Calories: 320
- Protein: 15g
- Carbohydrates: 50g
- Fat: 8g
- Fiber: 10g

Wild Rice with Mixed Mushrooms

- **Total Time:** 45 minutes
- **Servings:** 4

Ingredients:
- 1 cup wild rice, cooked
- 2 tablespoons olive oil
- 1 onion, diced
- 2 cloves garlic, minced
- 8 oz mixed mushrooms (shiitake, cremini, oyster), sliced
- 1 teaspoon thyme
- Salt and pepper to taste
- 1/4 cup fresh parsley, chopped
- Lemon wedges for serving

Directions:
1. In a skillet, heat olive oil and sauté onion until softened.
2. Add minced garlic and sliced mushrooms. Cook until mushrooms are golden brown.
3. Stir in cooked wild rice, thyme, salt, and pepper. Cook for an additional 5 minutes.
4. Garnish with fresh parsley and serve with lemon wedges.

Nutritional Information (per serving):
- Calories: 280
- Protein: 8g
- Carbohydrates: 40g
- Fat: 10g
- Fiber: 5g

Spicy Edamame Stir-Fry

- **Total Time:** 15 minutes
- **Servings:** 2

Ingredients:
- 2 cups edamame, shelled
- 1 cup broccoli florets
- 1 bell pepper, sliced
- 1 carrot, julienned

- 2 tablespoons soy sauce
- 1 tablespoon sriracha sauce
- 1 tablespoon sesame oil
- 1 tablespoon rice vinegar
- 1 tablespoon sesame seeds
- Green onions, chopped (for garnish)
- Cooked brown rice (for serving)

Directions:
1. In a wok or skillet, stir-fry edamame, broccoli, bell pepper, and carrot until vegetables are tender-crisp.
2. In a small bowl, whisk together soy sauce, sriracha sauce, sesame oil, and rice vinegar.
3. Pour the sauce over the vegetables and toss to coat.
4. Sprinkle sesame seeds and garnish with chopped green onions.
5. Serve over cooked brown rice.

Nutritional Information (per serving):
- Calories: 320
- Protein: 20g
- Carbohydrates: 30g
- Fat: 15g
- Fiber: 10g

Red Lentil Soup with Turmeric

- **Total Time:** 30 minutes
- **Servings:** 4

Ingredients:
- 1 cup red lentils, rinsed
- 1 onion, diced
- 2 carrots, diced
- 2 cloves garlic, minced
- 1 teaspoon ground turmeric
- 1 teaspoon ground cumin
- 6 cups vegetable broth
- 1 can (14 oz) diced tomatoes
- Salt and pepper to taste
- Fresh cilantro for garnish

Directions:

1. In a large pot, sauté onion and garlic until softened.
2. Add diced carrots, ground turmeric, ground cumin, and red lentils. Cook for 2 minutes.
3. Pour in vegetable broth and diced tomatoes. Bring to a simmer.
4. Cover and cook for 20-25 minutes or until lentils are tender.
5. Season with salt and pepper.
6. Garnish with fresh cilantro before serving.

Nutritional Information (per serving):

- Calories: 280
- Protein: 15g
- Carbohydrates: 50g
- Fat: 2g
- Fiber: 15g

Nuts and Seeds

Walnut-Crusted Salmon

- **Total Time:** 20 minutes
- **Servings:** 2

Ingredients:
- 2 salmon fillets
- 1/2 cup walnuts, finely chopped
- 2 tablespoons Dijon mustard
- 1 tablespoon honey
- 1 tablespoon olive oil
- Salt and pepper to taste
- Lemon wedges for serving

Directions:
1. Preheat the oven to 400°F (200°C).
2. In a bowl, mix chopped walnuts, Dijon mustard, honey, olive oil, salt, and pepper.
3. Place salmon fillets on a baking sheet lined with parchment paper.
4. Spread the walnut mixture over the salmon.
5. Bake for 12-15 minutes or until the salmon is cooked through.
6. Serve with lemon wedges.

Nutritional Information (per serving):
- Calories: 320
- Protein: 25g
- Carbohydrates: 8g
- Fat: 20g
- Fiber: 2g

Almond-Crusted Chicken Tenders

- **Total Time:** 25 minutes
- **Servings:** 3

Ingredients:
- 1 pound chicken tenders
- 1 cup almonds, finely ground
- 1 teaspoon paprika

- 1 teaspoon garlic powder
- Salt and pepper to taste
- 2 eggs, beaten
- Olive oil for cooking
- Greek yogurt or honey mustard for dipping

Directions:
1. Preheat the oven to 400°F (200°C).
2. In a bowl, mix ground almonds, paprika, garlic powder, salt, and pepper.
3. Dip each chicken tender into beaten eggs, then coat with the almond mixture.
4. Place the coated tenders on a baking sheet.
5. Drizzle with olive oil and bake for 15-20 minutes or until golden and cooked through.
6. Serve with Greek yogurt or honey mustard for dipping.

Nutritional Information (per serving):
- Calories: 280
- Protein: 30g
- Carbohydrates: 6g
- Fat: 15g
- Fiber: 4g

Pecan-Crusted Tilapia

- **Total Time:** 20 minutes
- **Servings:** 4

Ingredients:
- 4 tilapia fillets
- 1 cup pecans, finely chopped
- 1/4 cup whole wheat flour
- 1 teaspoon smoked paprika
- Salt and pepper to taste
- 2 tablespoons Dijon mustard
- Olive oil for cooking
- Fresh parsley for garnish
- Lemon wedges for serving

Directions:
1. In a shallow dish, combine chopped pecans, whole wheat flour, smoked paprika, salt, and pepper.

2. Brush each tilapia fillet with Dijon mustard.
3. Dredge the fillets in the pecan mixture, pressing gently to adhere.
4. Heat olive oil in a skillet over medium heat.
5. Cook tilapia fillets for 3-4 minutes per side or until golden and cooked through.
6. Garnish with fresh parsley and serve with lemon wedges.

Nutritional Information (per serving):
- Calories: 320
- Protein: 25g
- Carbohydrates: 8g
- Fat: 20g
- Fiber: 3g

Pistachio-Crusted Cod

- **Total Time:** 25 minutes
- **Servings:** 2

Ingredients:
- 2 cod fillets
- 1/2 cup pistachios, finely chopped
- 2 tablespoons whole wheat flour
- 1 teaspoon lemon zest
- Salt and pepper to taste
- 2 tablespoons plain Greek yogurt
- 1 tablespoon Dijon mustard
- Olive oil for cooking
- Lemon wedges for serving

Directions:
1. Preheat the oven to 400°F (200°C).
2. In a bowl, mix chopped pistachios, whole wheat flour, lemon zest, salt, and pepper.
3. In a separate bowl, combine Greek yogurt and Dijon mustard.
4. Brush each cod fillet with the yogurt-mustard mixture.
5. Dredge the fillets in the pistachio mixture, pressing gently to adhere.
6. Heat olive oil in an oven-safe skillet over medium-high heat.
7. Cook cod fillets for 2-3 minutes per side, then transfer the skillet to the oven.
8. Bake for an additional 10-12 minutes or until the cod is cooked through.
9. Serve with lemon wedges.

Nutritional Information (per serving):
- Calories: 280
- Protein: 30g
- Carbohydrates: 10g
- Fat: 15g
- Fiber: 3g

Sesame-Crusted Tofu

- **Total Time:** 30 minutes
- **Servings:** 3

Ingredients:
- 1 block extra-firm tofu, pressed and sliced
- 1/2 cup sesame seeds
- 2 tablespoons soy sauce
- 1 tablespoon rice vinegar
- 1 teaspoon sesame oil
- 1 teaspoon honey
- 1 teaspoon grated ginger
- Green onions for garnish
- Cooked brown rice (for serving)

Directions:
1. Preheat the oven to 400°F (200°C).
2. Press sliced tofu between paper towels to remove excess moisture.
3. Dip each tofu slice into soy sauce, then coat with sesame seeds.
4. Place the sesame-crusted tofu on a baking sheet.
5. Bake for 20-25 minutes or until golden and crispy.
6. In a bowl, whisk together soy sauce, rice vinegar, sesame oil, honey, and grated ginger.
7. Drizzle the sauce over the baked tofu.
8. Garnish with chopped green onions.
9. Serve over cooked brown rice.

Nutritional Information (per serving):
- Calories: 280
- Protein: 15g
- Carbohydrates: 15g
- Fat: 18g
- Fiber: 5g

Chia Seed Energy Balls

- **Total Time:** 15 minutes
- **Servings:** 12 balls

Ingredients:
- 1 cup rolled oats
- 1/2 cup almond butter
- 1/3 cup honey or maple syrup
- 1/4 cup chia seeds
- 1/4 cup ground flaxseeds
- 1/2 cup dark chocolate chips
- 1 teaspoon vanilla extract
- A pinch of salt

Directions:
1. In a bowl, combine rolled oats, almond butter, honey or maple syrup, chia seeds, ground flaxseeds, chocolate chips, vanilla extract, and a pinch of salt.
2. Mix until well combined.
3. Chill the mixture in the refrigerator for 30 minutes.
4. Once chilled, roll the mixture into bite-sized balls.
5. Store in an airtight container in the refrigerator.

Nutritional Information (per serving - 1 ball):
- Calories: 120
- Protein: 3g
- Carbohydrates: 14g
- Fat: 7g
- Fiber: 2g

Sunflower Seed-Crusted Chicken

- **Total Time:** 25 minutes
- **Servings:** 4

Ingredients:
- 4 boneless, skinless chicken breasts
- 1/2 cup sunflower seeds, finely ground
- 2 tablespoons Dijon mustard
- 1 tablespoon olive oil
- Salt and pepper to taste
- Lemon wedges for serving

Directions:

1. Preheat the oven to 400°F (200°C).
2. In a shallow dish, mix ground sunflower seeds, Dijon mustard, olive oil, salt, and pepper.
3. Coat each chicken breast with the sunflower seed mixture.
4. Place the coated chicken breasts on a baking sheet.
5. Bake for 20-25 minutes or until the chicken is cooked through.
6. Serve with lemon wedges.

Nutritional Information (per serving):

- Calories: 280
- Protein: 30g
- Carbohydrates: 2g
- Fat: 18g
- Fiber: 1g

Pumpkin Seed Pesto Pasta

- **Total Time:** 30 minutes
- **Servings:** 4

Ingredients:

- 8 oz whole wheat pasta
- 1 cup pumpkin seeds (pepitas), toasted
- 2 cups fresh basil leaves
- 1/2 cup grated Parmesan cheese
- 1/2 cup olive oil
- 2 cloves garlic
- Salt and pepper to taste
- Cherry tomatoes for garnish

Directions:

1. Cook pasta according to package instructions.
2. In a food processor, blend toasted pumpkin seeds, basil, Parmesan cheese, garlic, salt, and pepper.
3. While blending, gradually add olive oil until the pesto reaches a smooth consistency.
4. Toss cooked pasta with the pumpkin seed pesto.
5. Garnish with cherry tomatoes.

Nutritional Information (per serving):
- Calories: 480
- Protein: 15g
- Carbohydrates: 40g
- Fat: 30g
- Fiber: 6g

Cashew and Broccoli Stir-Fry

- **Total Time:** 20 minutes
- **Servings:** 3

Ingredients:
- 2 cups broccoli florets
- 1 cup cashews
- 1 pound tofu, cubed
- 2 tablespoons soy sauce
- 1 tablespoon hoisin sauce
- 1 tablespoon sesame oil
- 1 tablespoon olive oil
- 2 cloves garlic, minced
- Cooked brown rice (for serving)

Directions:
1. In a wok or skillet, heat olive oil and sauté garlic until fragrant.
2. Add tofu and stir-fry until golden.
3. Add broccoli and cashews to the wok.
4. In a small bowl, mix soy sauce, hoisin sauce, and sesame oil. Pour the sauce over the stir-fry.
5. Stir-fry until the broccoli is tender-crisp.
6. Serve over cooked brown rice.

Nutritional Information (per serving):
- Calories: 420
- Protein: 20g
- Carbohydrates: 25g
- Fat: 30g
- Fiber: 5g

Flaxseed and Berry Smoothie

- **Total Time:** 10 minutes
- **Servings:** 2

Ingredients:
- 1 cup mixed berries (strawberries, blueberries, raspberries)
- 1 banana
- 2 tablespoons ground flaxseeds
- 1 cup Greek yogurt
- 1 cup almond milk
- Honey or maple syrup to taste (optional)
- Ice cubes (optional)

Directions:
1. In a blender, combine mixed berries, banana, ground flaxseeds, Greek yogurt, and almond milk.
2. Blend until smooth.
3. Sweeten with honey or maple syrup if desired.
4. Add ice cubes and blend again for a chilled smoothie.
5. Pour into glasses and enjoy.

Nutritional Information (per serving):
- Calories: 250
- Protein: 12g
- Carbohydrates: 35g
- Fat: 8g
- Fiber: 8g

Snacks

Greek Yogurt and Cucumber Dip

- **Total Time:** 10 minutes
- **Servings:** 4

Ingredients:

- 1 cup Greek yogurt
- 1 cucumber, finely diced
- 2 tablespoons fresh dill, chopped
- 1 clove garlic, minced
- Salt and pepper to taste
- Olive oil for drizzling

Directions:

1. In a bowl, combine Greek yogurt, diced cucumber, chopped dill, minced garlic, salt, and pepper.
2. Mix until well combined.
3. Drizzle with olive oil before serving.
4. Serve with whole grain pita chips or vegetable sticks.

Nutritional Information (per serving):

- Calories: 80
- Protein: 5g
- Carbohydrates: 6g
- Fat: 4g
- Fiber: 1g

Hummus and Veggie Sticks

- **Total Time:** 15 minutes
- **Servings:** 4

Ingredients:

- 1 cup hummus
- Carrot sticks
- Cucumber sticks
- Bell pepper strips
- Cherry tomatoes

Directions:

1. Arrange hummus in a serving bowl.
2. Prepare carrot sticks, cucumber sticks, bell pepper strips, and cherry tomatoes.
3. Serve the veggie sticks alongside the hummus for dipping.
4. Enjoy this nutritious and satisfying snack.

Nutritional Information (per serving):

- Calories: 150
- Protein: 6g
- Carbohydrates: 20g
- Fat: 7g
- Fiber: 6g

Trail Mix with Dried Fruits and Nuts

- **Total Time:** 5 minutes
- **Servings:** 6

Ingredients:

- 1 cup mixed nuts (almonds, walnuts, cashews)
- 1/2 cup dried cranberries
- 1/2 cup dried apricots, chopped
- 1/4 cup dark chocolate chips
- 1/4 cup pumpkin seeds

Directions:

1. In a bowl, mix together mixed nuts, dried cranberries, chopped dried apricots, dark chocolate chips, and pumpkin seeds.
2. Toss until well combined.
3. Portion into individual servings for a quick and portable snack.

Nutritional Information (per serving):

- Calories: 200
- Protein: 5g
- Carbohydrates: 20g
- Fat: 12g
- Fiber: 4g

Roasted Chickpeas with Spices

- **Total Time:** 40 minutes
- **Servings:** 4

Ingredients:
- 2 cans (15 oz each) chickpeas, drained and rinsed
- 2 tablespoons olive oil
- 1 teaspoon ground cumin
- 1 teaspoon smoked paprika
- 1/2 teaspoon garlic powder
- 1/2 teaspoon cayenne pepper (optional)
- Salt to taste

Directions:
1. Preheat the oven to 400°F (200°C).
2. In a bowl, toss chickpeas with olive oil, ground cumin, smoked paprika, garlic powder, cayenne pepper (if using), and salt.
3. Spread chickpeas in a single layer on a baking sheet.
4. Roast for 30-35 minutes or until chickpeas are crispy, shaking the pan halfway through.
5. Allow to cool before serving.

Nutritional Information (per serving):
- Calories: 180
- Protein: 7g
- Carbohydrates: 25g
- Fat: 6g
- Fiber: 6g

Apple Slices with Almond Butter

- **Total Time:** 5 minutes
- **Servings:** 2

Ingredients:
- 2 apples, sliced
- 1/4 cup almond butter
- Cinnamon for sprinkling (optional)

Directions:
1. Slice the apples into thin wedges.
2. Spread almond butter on each apple slice.
3. Sprinkle with cinnamon if desired.
4. Enjoy this simple and satisfying snack.

Nutritional Information (per serving):
- Calories: 200
- Protein: 4g
- Carbohydrates: 25g
- Fat: 12g
- Fiber: 6g

Cottage Cheese and Pineapple Salsa

- **Total Time:** 10 minutes
- **Servings:** 2

Ingredients:
- 1 cup cottage cheese
- 1 cup fresh pineapple, diced
- 1/4 cup red bell pepper, finely chopped
- 2 tablespoons red onion, finely chopped
- 1 tablespoon fresh cilantro, chopped
- Salt and pepper to taste

Directions:
1. In a bowl, combine cottage cheese, diced pineapple, chopped red bell pepper, red onion, and cilantro.
2. Season with salt and pepper to taste.
3. Mix well and serve chilled.
4. Enjoy with whole grain crackers or as a refreshing dip.

Nutritional Information (per serving):
- Calories: 160
- Protein: 12g
- Carbohydrates: 18g
- Fat: 5g
- Fiber: 2g

Guacamole with Whole Grain Tortilla Chips

- **Total Time:** 15 minutes
- **Servings:** 4

Ingredients:

- 3 ripe avocados
- 1 tomato, diced
- 1/4 cup red onion, finely chopped
- 1 clove garlic, minced
- 1 lime, juiced
- Salt and pepper to taste
- Whole grain tortilla chips for serving

Directions:

1. In a bowl, mash the avocados with a fork.
2. Add diced tomato, chopped red onion, minced garlic, lime juice, salt, and pepper.
3. Mix until well combined.
4. Serve with whole grain tortilla chips for a wholesome and delicious snack.

Nutritional Information (per serving):

- Calories: 180
- Protein: 4g
- Carbohydrates: 15g
- Fat: 14g
- Fiber: 7g

Edamame with Sea Salt

- **Total Time:** 5 minutes
- **Servings:** 2

Ingredients:

- 2 cups edamame (frozen, pre-cooked)
- Sea salt to taste

Directions:

1. Steam or microwave edamame according to package instructions.
2. Sprinkle it with sea salt to taste.
3. Toss to coat evenly.
4. Serve as a quick and nutritious snack.

Nutritional Information (per serving):
- Calories: 160
- Protein: 14g
- Carbohydrates: 10g
- Fat: 8g
- Fiber: 7g

Cherry Tomatoes with Mozzarella

- **Total Time:** 10 minutes
- **Servings:** 2

Ingredients:
- 1 cup cherry tomatoes
- 1/2 cup fresh mozzarella balls
- Fresh basil leaves
- Balsamic glaze for drizzling

Directions:
1. Thread cherry tomatoes, fresh mozzarella balls, and basil leaves onto toothpicks.
2. Arrange the skewers on a serving plate.
3. Drizzle with balsamic glaze just before serving.
4. Enjoy this delightful and colorful snack.

Nutritional Information (per serving):
- Calories: 180
- Protein: 10g
- Carbohydrates: 5g
- Fat: 14g
- Fiber: 1g

Greek Yogurt Parfait with Granola

- **Total Time:** 5 minutes
- **Servings:** 1

Ingredients:
- 1 cup Greek yogurt
- 1/2 cup granola
- 1/2 cup mixed berries (strawberries, blueberries, raspberries)
- Honey for drizzling (optional)

Directions:

1. In a glass or bowl, layer Greek yogurt, granola, and mixed berries.
2. Repeat the layers until the container is filled.
3. Drizzle with honey if desired.
4. Indulge in this tasty and protein-packed parfait.

Nutritional Information (per serving):

- Calories: 350
- Protein: 20g
- Carbohydrates: 40g
- Fat: 15g
- Fiber: 6g

Desserts

Berry and Yogurt Popsicles

- **Total Time:** 4 hours (including freezing time)
- **Servings:** 6

Ingredients:
- 1 cup mixed berries (strawberries, blueberries, raspberries)
- 1 cup Greek yogurt
- 2 tablespoons honey
- 1 teaspoon vanilla extract

Directions:
1. In a blender, combine mixed berries, Greek yogurt, honey, and vanilla extract.
2. Blend until smooth.
3. Pour the mixture into popsicle molds.
4. Insert popsicle sticks and freeze for at least 4 hours or until solid.
5. Enjoy these refreshing and healthy popsicles.

Nutritional Information (per serving):
- Calories: 80
- Protein: 5g
- Carbohydrates: 15g
- Fat: 1g
- Fiber: 2g

Dark Chocolate and Almond Clusters

- **Total Time:** 20 minutes
- **Servings:** 12 clusters

Ingredients:
- 1 cup dark chocolate chips
- 1 cup almonds, whole or chopped
- Sea salt for sprinkling (optional)

Directions:
1. Melt dark chocolate chips in a microwave-safe bowl or using a double boiler.
2. Stir in almonds until well coated.

3. Spoon small clusters of the mixture onto a parchment-lined tray.
4. Sprinkle with sea salt if desired.
5. Allow to cool and harden at room temperature or in the refrigerator.
6. Indulge in these sweet and nutty chocolate clusters.

Nutritional Information (per serving - 1 cluster):
- Calories: 90
- Protein: 2g
- Carbohydrates: 8g
- Fat: 6g
- Fiber: 2g

Baked Apples with Cinnamon and Walnuts

- **Total Time:** 40 minutes
- **Servings:** 4

Ingredients:
- 4 apples, cored and halved
- 1/4 cup chopped walnuts
- 2 tablespoons honey or maple syrup
- 1 teaspoon ground cinnamon
- Greek yogurt for serving (optional)

Directions:
1. Preheat the oven to 375°F (190°C).
2. Place apple halves in a baking dish.
3. In a bowl, mix chopped walnuts, honey or maple syrup, and ground cinnamon.
4. Spoon the mixture into the center of each apple half.
5. Bake for 30-35 minutes or until the apples are tender.
6. Serve with a dollop of Greek yogurt if desired.
7. Enjoy this warm and comforting dessert.

Nutritional Information (per serving):
- Calories: 150
- Protein: 2g
- Carbohydrates: 30g
- Fat: 5g
- Fiber: 5g

Avocado Chocolate Mousse

- **Total Time:** 15 minutes
- **Servings:** 4

Ingredients:
- 2 ripe avocados
- 1/2 cup unsweetened cocoa powder
- 1/2 cup almond milk
- 1/4 cup maple syrup or agave nectar
- 1 teaspoon vanilla extract
- A pinch of salt
- Fresh berries for garnish

Directions:
1. Scoop the flesh of avocados into a blender.
2. Add cocoa powder, almond milk, maple syrup or agave nectar, vanilla extract, and a pinch of salt.
3. Blend until smooth and creamy.
4. Spoon into serving dishes and refrigerate for at least 1 hour.
5. Garnish with fresh berries before serving.
6. Delight in this rich and guilt-free chocolate mousse.

Nutritional Information (per serving):
- Calories: 220
- Protein: 3g
- Carbohydrates: 22g
- Fat: 15g
- Fiber: 7g

Mango Sorbet with Mint

- **Total Time:** 4 hours (including freezing time)
- **Servings:** 4

Ingredients:
- 2 cups ripe mango, diced
- 1/4 cup fresh mint leaves
- 1/4 cup honey or agave nectar
- 1 tablespoon lime juice
- 1/2 cup water

Directions:

1. In a blender, combine diced mango, mint leaves, honey or agave nectar, lime juice, and water.
2. Blend until smooth.
3. Pour the mixture into a shallow dish and freeze for at least 4 hours, stirring every hour for a smoother texture.
4. Scoop into bowls and garnish with additional mint leaves.
5. Enjoy this fruity and refreshing mango sorbet.

Nutritional Information (per serving):

- Calories: 120
- Protein: 1g
- Carbohydrates: 30g
- Fat: 0g
- Fiber: 2g

Poached Pears in Red Wine

- **Total Time:** 1 hour
- **Servings:** 4

Ingredients:

- 4 ripe but firm pears, peeled and cored
- 1 bottle red wine
- 1 cup water
- 1 cup granulated sugar
- 1 cinnamon stick
- 1 orange, zest and juice
- Vanilla ice cream for serving (optional)

Directions:

1. In a large pot, combine red wine, water, sugar, cinnamon stick, orange zest, and juice.
2. Bring the mixture to a simmer over medium heat.
3. Add the peeled and cored pears, ensuring they are fully submerged.
4. Simmer for 30-40 minutes or until pears are tender, turning occasionally.
5. Remove the pears and let the poaching liquid reduce for another 10 minutes.
6. Serve the poached pears with the reduced wine sauce.
7. Optionally, serve with a scoop of vanilla ice cream.

Nutritional Information (per serving):
- Calories: 300
- Protein: 1g
- Carbohydrates: 60g
- Fat: 0g
- Fiber: 5g

Greek Yogurt Cheesecake with Berry Compote

- **Total Time:** 4 hours (including chilling time)
- **Servings:** 8

Ingredients:

For the Cheesecake:
- 2 cups Greek yogurt
- 1 cup cream cheese
- 1/2 cup honey
- 1 teaspoon vanilla extract
- 3 large eggs

For the Berry Compote:
- 2 cups mixed berries (strawberries, blueberries, raspberries)
- 2 tablespoons honey
- 1 tablespoon lemon juice

Directions:

For the Cheesecake:
1. Preheat the oven to 325°F (163°C).
2. In a bowl, combine Greek yogurt, cream cheese, honey, vanilla extract, and eggs.
3. Mix until smooth and creamy.
4. Pour the mixture into a prepared crust or a springform pan.
5. Bake for 40-45 minutes or until the center is set.
6. Let it cool and refrigerate for at least 3 hours.

For the Berry Compote:
1. In a saucepan, combine mixed berries, honey, and lemon juice.
2. Simmer over low heat until the berries break down and the mixture thickens.
3. Let it cool before serving over the cheesecake.

Nutritional Information (per serving):
- Calories: 350
- Protein: 12g
- Carbohydrates: 30g

- Fat: 20g
- Fiber: 3g

Pumpkin Pie Oat Bars

- **Total Time:** 45 minutes
- **Servings:** 12

Ingredients:
- 2 cups rolled oats
- 1 cup canned pumpkin
- 1/2 cup almond butter
- 1/4 cup maple syrup
- 1 teaspoon pumpkin pie spice
- 1/2 teaspoon vanilla extract
- A pinch of salt
- 1/4 cup chocolate chips (optional)

Directions:
1. Preheat the oven to 350°F (175°C) and line a baking dish with parchment paper.
2. In a bowl, combine rolled oats, canned pumpkin, almond butter, maple syrup, pumpkin pie spice, vanilla extract, and a pinch of salt.
3. Mix until well combined.
4. Press the mixture into the prepared baking dish.
5. Sprinkle chocolate chips on top if desired.
6. Bake for 25-30 minutes or until the edges are golden.
7. Allow to cool before slicing into bars.

Nutritional Information (per serving):
- Calories: 150
- Protein: 4g
- Carbohydrates: 20g
- Fat: 7g
- Fiber: 3g

Coconut and Date Energy Bites

- **Total Time:** 15 minutes
- **Servings:** 16

Ingredients:
- 1 cup shredded coconut
- 1 cup dates, pitted
- 1/2 cup almonds
- 1/4 cup cocoa powder
- 1 tablespoon coconut oil
- 1 teaspoon vanilla extract
- A pinch of salt

Directions:
1. In a food processor, combine shredded coconut, dates, almonds, cocoa powder, coconut oil, vanilla extract, and a pinch of salt.
2. Process until the mixture forms a sticky dough.
3. Roll the dough into bite-sized balls.
4. Refrigerate for at least 30 minutes before serving.

Nutritional Information (per serving):
- Calories: 80
- Protein: 1g
- Carbohydrates: 10g
- Fat: 5g
- Fiber: 2g

Grilled Pineapple with Honey and Pistachios

- **Total Time:** 15 minutes
- **Servings:** 4

Ingredients:
- 1 pineapple, peeled, cored, and sliced
- 2 tablespoons honey
- 1/4 cup pistachios, chopped
- Fresh mint leaves for garnish (optional)

Directions:
1. Preheat the grill to medium-high heat.

2. Grill the pineapple slices for 2-3 minutes on each side or until grill marks appear.
3. Drizzle honey over the grilled pineapple slices.
4. Sprinkle chopped pistachios on top.
5. Garnish with fresh mint leaves if desired.
6. Serve immediately and enjoy this simple and delightful grilled dessert.

Nutritional Information (per serving):
- Calories: 120
- Protein: 2g
- Carbohydrates: 28g
- Fat: 2g
- Fiber: 3g

Smoothies

Berry Blast Smoothie with Spinach

- **Total Time:** 5 minutes
- **Servings:** 2

Ingredients:

- 1 cup mixed berries (strawberries, blueberries, raspberries)
- 1 banana
- 1 cup spinach leaves
- 1/2 cup Greek yogurt
- 1 cup almond milk
- Ice cubes (optional)

Directions:

1. In a blender, combine mixed berries, banana, spinach leaves, Greek yogurt, and almond milk.
2. Blend until smooth.
3. Add ice cubes if desired and blend again.
4. Pour into glasses and enjoy this nutrient-packed berry and spinach smoothie.

Nutritional Information (per serving):

- Calories: 150
- Protein: 7g
- Carbohydrates: 30g
- Fat: 2g
- Fiber: 6g

Green Tea and Mango Smoothie

- **Total Time:** 7 minutes
- **Servings:** 2

Ingredients:

- 1 cup brewed green tea, cooled
- 1 cup frozen mango chunks
- 1 banana
- 1 tablespoon chia seeds
- 1/2 cup plain Greek yogurt

- Honey or agave nectar to taste
- Ice cubes (optional)

Directions:
1. Brew green tea and let it cool to room temperature.
2. In a blender, combine green tea, frozen mango chunks, banana, chia seeds, and Greek yogurt.
3. Add honey or agave nectar to sweeten, if desired.
4. Blend until smooth.
5. Add ice cubes if you want a colder consistency.
6. Pour into glasses and savor this refreshing green tea and mango smoothie.

Nutritional Information (per serving):
- Calories: 180
- Protein: 8g
- Carbohydrates: 35g
- Fat: 3g
- Fiber: 6g

Pineapple and Kale Smoothie

- **Total Time:** 6 minutes
- **Servings:** 2

Ingredients:
- 1 cup fresh pineapple chunks
- 1 cup kale leaves, stems removed
- 1 banana
- 1/2 cup coconut water
- 1/2 cup almond milk
- 1 tablespoon flaxseeds
- Ice cubes (optional)

Directions:
1. In a blender, combine fresh pineapple chunks, kale leaves, banana, coconut water, almond milk, and flaxseeds.
2. Blend until smooth.
3. Add ice cubes for a colder consistency if desired.
4. Pour into glasses and relish this tropical pineapple and kale smoothie.

Nutritional Information (per serving):
- Calories: 160
- Protein: 5g
- Carbohydrates: 30g
- Fat: 4g
- Fiber: 7g

Blueberry and Almond Milk Smoothie

- **Total Time:** 5 minutes
- **Servings:** 2

Ingredients:
- 1 cup blueberries (fresh or frozen)
- 1 banana
- 1 cup almond milk
- 1/2 cup Greek yogurt
- 2 tablespoons almond butter
- 1 teaspoon honey (optional)
- Ice cubes (optional)

Directions:
1. In a blender, combine blueberries, banana, almond milk, Greek yogurt, almond butter, and honey if desired.
2. Blend until smooth.
3. Add ice cubes for a chilled and refreshing texture.
4. Pour into glasses and enjoy this delicious blueberry and almond milk smoothie.

Nutritional Information (per serving):
- Calories: 200
- Protein: 8g
- Carbohydrates: 30g
- Fat: 7g
- Fiber: 6g

Banana and Peanut Butter Protein Smoothie

- **Total Time:** 6 minutes
- **Servings:** 2

Ingredients:
- 2 ripe bananas
- 2 tablespoons peanut butter
- 1 cup milk (dairy or plant-based)
- 1/2 cup Greek yogurt
- 1 scoop protein powder (vanilla or chocolate)
- Ice cubes (optional)

Directions:
1. In a blender, combine ripe bananas, peanut butter, milk, Greek yogurt, and protein powder.
2. Blend until smooth.
3. Add ice cubes if you prefer a colder consistency.
4. Pour into glasses and enjoy this protein-packed banana and peanut butter smoothie.

Nutritional Information (per serving):
- Calories: 300
- Protein: 20g
- Carbohydrates: 35g
- Fat: 12g
- Fiber: 4g

Spinach and Pineapple Detox Smoothie

- **Total Time:** 5 minutes
- **Servings:** 2

Ingredients:
- 2 cups fresh spinach leaves
- 1 cup pineapple chunks (fresh or frozen)
- 1 banana
- 1/2 cucumber, peeled and sliced
- 1 tablespoon chia seeds
- 1 cup coconut water
- Ice cubes (optional)

Directions:

1. In a blender, combine fresh spinach leaves, pineapple chunks, banana, cucumber, chia seeds, and coconut water.
2. Blend until smooth.
3. Add ice cubes for a refreshing chill.
4. Pour into glasses and enjoy this detoxifying spinach and pineapple smoothie.

Nutritional Information (per serving):

- Calories: 120
- Protein: 3g
- Carbohydrates: 25g
- Fat: 2g
- Fiber: 6g

Avocado and Berry Smoothie

- **Total Time:** 6 minutes
- **Servings:** 2

Ingredients:

- 1 ripe avocado
- 1 cup mixed berries (strawberries, blueberries, raspberries)
- 1 banana
- 1 cup almond milk
- 1 tablespoon honey
- 1/2 teaspoon vanilla extract
- Ice cubes (optional)

Directions:

1. In a blender, combine ripe avocado, mixed berries, banana, almond milk, honey, and vanilla extract.
2. Blend until smooth.
3. Add ice cubes for a cooler texture.
4. Pour into glasses and savor the creamy goodness of this avocado and berry smoothie.

Nutritional Information (per serving):

- Calories: 250
- Protein: 4g
- Carbohydrates: 35g
- Fat: 12g
- Fiber: 8g

Watermelon and Mint Smoothie

- **Total Time:** 5 minutes
- **Servings:** 2

Ingredients:
- 2 cups fresh watermelon, diced
- 1/2 cup Greek yogurt
- 1 tablespoon fresh mint leaves
- 1 tablespoon lime juice
- 1 teaspoon honey
- Ice cubes (optional)

Directions:
1. In a blender, combine fresh watermelon, Greek yogurt, mint leaves, lime juice, and honey.
2. Blend until smooth.
3. Add ice cubes for a cooler and slushier consistency.
4. Pour into glasses and relish the refreshing taste of this watermelon and mint smoothie.

Nutritional Information (per serving):
- Calories: 100
- Protein: 5g
- Carbohydrates: 20g
- Fat: 1g
- Fiber: 1g

Kiwi and Orange Smoothie

- **Total Time:** 5 minutes
- **Servings:** 2

Ingredients:
- 3 kiwis, peeled and sliced
- 2 oranges, peeled and segmented
- 1 banana
- 1/2 cup plain Greek yogurt
- 1 tablespoon flaxseeds
- 1 cup orange juice
- Ice cubes (optional)

Directions:

1. In a blender, combine kiwis, oranges, banana, Greek yogurt, flaxseeds, and orange juice.
2. Blend until smooth.
3. Add ice cubes for a frosty texture.
4. Pour into glasses and enjoy the zesty goodness of this kiwi and orange smoothie.

Nutritional Information (per serving):

- Calories: 180
- Protein: 6g
- Carbohydrates: 40g
- Fat: 2g
- Fiber: 8g

Carrot and Ginger Immunity Boosting Smoothie

- **Total Time:** 7 minutes
- **Servings:** 2

Ingredients:

- 2 carrots, peeled and sliced
- 1 orange, peeled and segmented
- 1 banana
- 1-inch piece of ginger, peeled and grated
- 1 tablespoon chia seeds
- 1 cup coconut water
- Ice cubes (optional)

Directions:

1. In a blender, combine sliced carrots, orange segments, banana, grated ginger, chia seeds, and coconut water.
2. Blend until smooth.
3. Add ice cubes for a chilled and invigorating experience.
4. Pour into glasses and embrace the immune-boosting power of this carrot and ginger smoothie.

Nutritional Information (per serving):

- Calories: 140
- Protein: 3g
- Carbohydrates: 30g
- Fat: 2g
- Fiber: 7g

Conclusion

In the concluding chapters of our "Prostate Cancer Diet Cookbook for Men," it is paramount to reflect on the profound impact that nutrition can have on the well-being and health of the prostate. The journey you've embarked on, guided by wholesome and purposeful dietary choices, is a testament to the commitment you've shown to prioritize your health.

As you traverse the pages of this cookbook, it's essential to acknowledge the profound connection between nutrition and prostate health. The recipes meticulously crafted with ingredients rich in antioxidants, vitamins, and minerals have been specifically chosen to support and nourish the prostate. From the vibrant colors of fruits and vegetables to the lean proteins and whole grains, each ingredient plays a crucial role in promoting overall well-being.

The understanding that food is not merely sustenance but a powerful tool in fostering health is a key takeaway. Research suggests that certain nutrients and compounds found in our daily meals may contribute to the prevention and management of prostate cancer. Antioxidants, in particular, have been associated with reducing oxidative stress, potentially influencing the development and progression of prostate cancer.

Moreover, the incorporation of plant-based foods, lean proteins, and a variety of grains not only supports prostate health but contributes to your overall vitality. By adopting a balanced and diverse diet, you are not only nurturing your prostate but also fostering a robust immune system, maintaining a healthy weight, and promoting cardiovascular health.

As you close the chapter on this cookbook, let it be the beginning of a sustained commitment to a prostate-friendly lifestyle. The recipes provided are not just culinary delights but tools for empowerment, equipping you with the knowledge to make informed choices for your health.

Remember, your journey to prostate health is not a solitary endeavor. It involves a holistic approach encompassing regular exercise, stress management, and, importantly, routine health check-ups. Consultation with healthcare professionals remains pivotal, and these recipes serve as a complementary element to your overall health plan.

In the pursuit of a healthy future, allow these recipes to inspire creativity in your kitchen. Experiment with flavors, tweak recipes to suit your preferences, and share the joy of nutritious and delicious meals with loved ones. Building a supportive community around health-conscious choices can amplify the positive impact on everyone involved.

In conclusion, this cookbook is not merely a collection of recipes; it's a guide to cultivating a lifestyle that nurtures your well-being. As you savor the flavors of each dish, relish the knowledge that you are actively contributing to your prostate health. Let this journey be a celebration of good food, good health, and the resilience of the human spirit in embracing a future filled with vitality and wellness. Cheers to your journey to prostate health!

Made in the USA
Las Vegas, NV
15 August 2024

93882507R10050